The Practical Caregiver's Guide to Home Hospice: How to Help Someone You Love

SARA M. BARTON

Copyright © 2017 Sara M. Barton

Second Edition

All rights reserved.

ISBN: 1545428476
ISBN-13: 978-1545428474

DEDICATION

For you, Dad. Thanks for teaching me that no matter how unfair life is, you never give up; and if you're going to do something, do it right.

In memory of my mother, who was challenged in the last ten years of her life by multiple surgeries, a heart attack, diabetes, COPD, and felled by the final insult -- lung cancer.

CONTENTS

Preface	1
Part One -- The Practical Side of Home Hospice	3
Section One -- Home Hospice Care Essentials	4
Section Two -- Home Hospice Changes Everything	7
Section Three -- Practical home Hospice Caregiver Skills	9
Section Four -- Create a Home Hospice Command Center	11
Section Five -- Organize Home Life Structure	
Section Six -- Have a Caregiver Support Team	14
Section Seven -- Organize the Medical Care in Home Hospice	19
Section Eight -- During End-of-Life Care (Hospice)	24
Part Two -- The Heart and Soul of Hospice	28
Section Nine -- Hospice Is End-of-Life Caregiving	29
Part Three -- Heading Toward Death	34
Section Ten -- The Dying Process Changes Everything	35
Part Four -- The Toll of Hospice Caregiving	44

Section Eleven -- Hospice Caregiving Can Affect You	45
Part Five -- As the Ends Nears	51
Section Twelve -- Don't Be Alone When Your Loved One Dies	52
Part Six -- After the Caregiving	56
Section Thirteen -- Grief and Grieving	57
Part Seven -- The Empty Chair	61
Section Fourteen -- Coping with the Loss	62
Author Information	67

THE PRACTICAL CAREGIVER'S GUIDE TO HOME HOSPICE

PREFACE

There are three important rules for good family care:

1. Love is never enough. You can love someone utterly and completely, but without the right tools and education, you can fail as a caregiver.

2. You have to take care of yourself in order to be able to take care of your loved one. If you fail, there will be two people who need a caregiver -- you and your loved one!

3. What you don't know or understand can hurt you AND your loved one -- when you learn about what ails your loved one, you can also learn about what will make care better.

Believe in yourself. Believe that for every

problem there is at least one solution. Believe in family care -- there's no place like home. Direct your caregiving to meet your loved one's real needs. The rewards can be great.

Love really does make the world go around, but if you want a smoother ride, grease the wheels!

PART ONE: THE PRACTICAL SIDE OF HOSPICE

SECTION ONE -- HOME HOSPICE CARE ESSENTIALS

What kind of home hospice caregiver are you? Did you volunteer when you found out your loved one had a life-limiting illness? Did you get the job because there was no one else available? Do you feel overwhelmed and unable to cope? Do you feel hopeful that you can make your loved one comfortable in his or her final months, weeks, or days?

Home hospice is an important time for families. It's a chance to make the most of the opportunities left -- to finish unfinished business, to say the final goodbye to someone you love. A practical caregiver is an educated caregiver. The more you know and understand about home hospice care, the better the care you will give. Why? You will understand that you cannot make your loved one better, but you can make him or her feel better. Comfort is the key to success in home hospice care.

When families work together to provide home hospice care, it can be extremely rewarding and bonding. A cooperative effort can help your loved one to prepare for his or her final journey with a sense of peace and sometimes even relief that the long, hard struggle is ending.

Home hospice care is different from other kinds of home care. If you have been the family caregiver for your loved one, you've probably spent a lot of time running back and forth to doctors' offices or the hospital. Now it's likely that your loved one will spend the final days at home, in familiar surroundings. There will be people coming to the house to help care for your loved one. The hospice team will work to manage any of the pain or discomfort as your loved one's health deteriorates. The effort is directed at making your loved one as comfortable as possible.

Some things are inevitable as the body begins to break down, and these issues will be addressed by the home hospice team. In most cases, you will be doing a lot of the physical work in caring for your loved one, and the hospice team will help you to understand the stages as your loved one goes through them. In addition to medical support, hospice programs have social workers, chaplains, and volunteers to help you cope with the emotional and social aspects of caring for a dying person. The stress can sometimes be overwhelming, so it's important that you work with the hospice team to get the kind of support you need to do the job.

Caregiver's Tip – Don't Despair

Some family caregivers can find the challenges of providing hospice care nearly impossible, especially if there aren't a lot of family members, friends, or neighbors available to help, or if the physical demands of caregiving take more than they can provide. It's important to be creative in finding the kinds of resources that can help you get through it. It's also important to know that some paid help is often covered under your loved one's insurance plan.

SECTION TWO -- HOME HOSPICE CHANGES EVERYTHING

Experienced caregivers sometimes have difficulty transitioning into home hospice care. When you are used to providing care that is directed towards a cure, towards preventing problems, it can be hard to realize and accept that your loved one's body is beginning to break down. You may find that some medications and treatments for your loved one are no longer being used. You may also find your loved one is no longer interested in eating. It can be emotionally tough to accept that fact. Home hospice is a time of uncertainty, doubt, and worry for many families. The better you understand what your role is as a home hospice caregiver, the better able you will be to meet the challenges of making your loved one as comfortable as possible at the end of life.

Comfort is more than just a body without pain. It is a mind that no longer worries that family life will change for the worse after death or that death will be physically painful. It is a heart that is not heavy with grief or anger because life is ending with so much left to do and not enough time or energy to do it. A practical home hospice caregiver learns that helping a loved one find peace at the end of life is all about empowerment. Listen to your loved one -- understand what is important to him or her. How should the last months, weeks, and days be spent? What is on that "to do" list, and how can you help him or her get as much done, even as the body begins to deteriorate?

Good home hospice care is all about adapting your care to meet the rapidly changing needs of your loved one. Things can happen quickly or unexpectedly. If you stay focused on your goal to help your loved one have a peaceful death, you will concentrate on doing what can be done to provide comfort and compassion at the end of your loved one's death. You will do the best you can under the circumstances you and your loved one face. That is all any human being can do.

SECTION THREE -- PRACTICAL HOME HOSPICE CAREGIVER SKILLS

1. Organize your home hospice caregiving.

2. Recognize the human needs at the end of life.

3. Realize the need to include family and friends in the care plan.

4. Minimize the growing weaknesses.

5. Maximize the continued strengths.

6. Utilize hospice resources and education.

7. Make yourself take respite time.

Caregiver Tip – Direct the Home Hospice Experience to Benefit Your Loved One

Time is growing short by the time your loved

one is placed in hospice care. Flexibility and adaptability are critical in meeting the needs of a dying loved one. Always ask yourself one question when you are making a decision that affects your loved one – "Will I regret doing or not doing this down the road?"

SECTION FOUR -- CREATE A HOME HOSPICE COMMAND CENTER

In order to focus your home hospice caregiving, you will need to create your Caregiver Command Center. This is where you organize and store all things related to the care you provide.

Physical Records Keeping

You need one central location to keep all of the printed information on your loved one's medical, financial, insurance, and personal issues that you will be handling. This includes any notes and instructions provided to you by nurses.

For many patients, insurance coverage for hospice care is very different than "cure care". Check with your hospice team, so that you understand what is changing. You may find that medications that were previously denied are now covered, even over-the-counter medications.

Electronic Records Keeping

You may also want to create an electronic file on your computer for important information. (You may choose to take advantage of some of the many programs and apps available to caregivers that help them get medications organized. The costs vary for these, as do the features.)

Many hospice patients have limited activities outside the home. Your loved one may no longer go out for medical appointments due to mobility issues, or may have a hospice physician or nurse make house calls when needed. One of the biggest responsibilities for family caregivers is medication management, and there are several options for tracking electronically, from software to phone apps.

There may also be some issues that will surface after your loved one's death. Having an electronic record of what happened during hospice may be helpful.

Caregiver Tip – Start (Or Restart) Yourself Off On the Right Foot

If you don't already have one, take the time to set up your command center. Errors can occur when things get hectic or chaotic. You will need to have an organized base for your caregiving in order to track your loved one's medications, treatments, and any hospice team directions. It doesn't have to be a big command center, with fancy doodads and gizmos. It does have to work for you, so that you can stay focused on providing the best hospice care to your loved one that you can.

SECTION FIVE -- ORGANIZE HOME LIFE STRUCTURE

If you are new to the hospice situation, it's important for you not only to understand your loved one's needs for care, but the benefits of having a caregiver structure. The worst thing in the world that a well-meaning caregiver can do is to micromanage the hospice setting. Every human being needs to feel that life is worth living, even if that means making more of an effort. This is especially true in hospice care. Time is growing short. There are often unmet needs and unfulfilled dreams. It's important to recognize that hospice care changes everything.

1. Needs – You are the official care assistant.

Make a list of the things your loved one needs to

do to prepare for death. Discuss this. Take the time to observe your loved one. When it becomes emotionally overwhelming, take a step back. When he or she seems interested in sharing final wishes, thoughts, and directives, record the instructions. If your loved one is physically uncomfortable, work with the hospice team to change it for the better.

2. Strengths – You are the official skills optimizer.

Make a list of the things your loved one can do by himself or herself at this moment in time. These can be used to maintain a sense of self-worth in your loved one, even during hospice. The more you encourage the use of these strengths, the less dependent your loved one will feel upon you. Everyone wants to feel like a contributor, not a burden. (Remember that things can change and you may need to adapt tools and assistance to meet these needs.) Find ways to enable him or her to continue achieving. Let your loved one's voice be heard, whether it's to impart wisdom to the family or share stories of days gone by. Ask if you can record the conversations, either with audio or video, or write them down.

3. Activities – You are the official social coordinator.

Many hospice patients can still participate in

activities, so consider what is possible for your loved one. You may still get together for family gatherings, but keep it simple. Friends and neighbors may still come by, if your loved one agrees. If family members are having a hard time coping with their emotions, talk to your hospice team. There are social workers and bereavement counselors available to help any family member in need, even before your loved one dies. Remember that everyone's goal is to make your loved one as comfortable as possible. People who are having trouble managing their emotions may wish to use alternative means of communication, sending cards and letters to show their support. In some cases, children and/or your loved one may not mutually benefit from visits, but certainly there are ways that children can share the love they feel, through drawings and other special projects that can be shared with your loved one.

Noise can trigger distress for hospice patients -- whether it's a scary movie on the TV, a barking dog, or a loud visitor of any age. Always pay attention to the needs of your loved one and make his or her comfort your priority. It's also important to know that even while sleeping, your loved one can hear what's going on in the hospice room. Loud conversations or rowdy music can disrupt your loved one's rest, even when no one thinks it matters.

Consider also the distress a hospice patient might feel upon hearing conversations that involve topics he or she might find upsetting.

4. Routines –You are the official domestic routines coordinator.

Make a list of the routines you need help doing while your loved one is in hospice care. Does the lawn need mowing? Does the driveway need shoveling so the nurse can attend to your loved one? Will you need to hire someone, call upon a family member or friend, or can you do it yourself? Don't stretch yourself too thin during hospice caregiving. As the main caregiver, you are the one responsible for your loved one. Use your resources to get things done. And don't be afraid to ask a family member to pitch in and help with the household responsibilities when you need to focus on hospice caregiving. That's what a team is for -- to get it all done right.

5. Schedules – You are the official schedule coordinator.

Make a list of the schedule your loved one normally keeps, so that you can keep things consistent and calm. What time does he or she usually get up? What time does he or she normally sleep or rest? When are meals usually eaten? When are medications taken? By following his or her normal schedule, you can help bring focus and a sense of normalcy to your loved one's life. You won't always be able to do things on schedule, but understanding it can be very helpful for everyone. Whether it's a visit from a friend or the dispensing of a medication, your loved one will be better able to handle it when it doesn't come at a low point in your loved one's day.

SECTION SIX -- HAVE A CAREGIVER SUPPORT TEAM

What is your caregiver support team? This is a critical issue for you to understand because your caregiver support team will help you avoid some of the biggest pitfalls of taking care of a loved one at the end of life. Stress, depression, and physical neglect can take its toll on family caregivers. The better you understand your responsibility to take good care of yourself, the better the care you will provide to your loved one. You need to be able to focus, to manage crises that arise, and to meet the constantly changing demands of caregiving. You will need:

1. Physical Support – You need help to get it all done.

You should never do hospice caregiving all by yourself. You need to know who you can call on for those times you need help providing care. Make a list of the people you can count on, what they can provide, and what their strengths are. There may be some people who are good at visiting your loved one when you want to pop out to the store for a few things. There may be others who are willing to be involved in regularly helping you with your loved one or things you need to have done. And remember to respect your loved one's needs when arranging for people to sit with him or her. Don't bring in someone who upsets your loved one by chattering too much or who can't handle the changes in your loved one. Invite people who are calm, confident, and caring to visit.

2. Emotional Support – You need a shoulder or two to cry on.

You will need emotional support during your time as a hospice caregiver, and the harder the challenges you face, the greater the need for quality support. Consider people who have walked in your shoes as family caregivers, because they know what it's like. It's especially important for you to reach out to your inner circle, so you feel connected to life while your loved one is dying. It helps to have good people on your team to help you troubleshoot issues and apply realistic solutions to problems. Avoid pessimistic people for your support team. Pessimists will bring you down at a point where you most need positive energy.

3. Financial/Work Support – You need help

balancing out the realities of caregiving.

If you are still working full-time when you take on the care of your loved one, you will need to work out the challenges of sometimes being in two places at once. If your loved one's physical needs require you to scale back your job to take on full-time caregiver duties, how will you manage the financial burdens of caring for your loved one?

Some families provide a stipend to family members providing care, to help cover the loss of wages. Caregivers still need to have medical and other insurances, but in some cases, it's possible to downsize temporarily. Make a list of your financial needs during hospice, consider ways to adjust them to fit the caregiver situation, and eliminate unnecessary costs.

Some people are able to work from home, and this can be an especially appealing choice during hospice. If your loved one is resting comfortably, you may be able get things done with a virtual office. If you make phone or conference calls, or hold business meetings, do it in another room, to avoid disturbing your loved one. Ask a family member, friend, neighbor, or a paid companion to sit with your loved one while you handle your duties from your virtual office.

You may choose to take a paid or unpaid leave in order to spend time with your loved one before that final good-bye. Some people are able to use their vacation time to cover some of their absence from work.

If you are having a difficult time juggling work

and hospice care, it's sometimes possible to partner with other family members, friends, and neighbors to provide coverage. You may also hire an experienced health care aide to be with your loved one during certain hours, if it is covered by insurance or you can afford this. A team approach can help you overcome some of the obstacles in juggling work and hospice.

4. Respite Care Support – Taking time for you is NOT optional!

Hospice caregivers need to understand and appreciate the critical need for respite care for themselves. Respite time allows you to recharge your batteries. You should never feel guilty. You are at a very emotional time in your life and you need some space from the hospice situation to compose yourself and process your emotions. Make a list of family members, friends, and neighbors you can call upon. Your hospice program has trained volunteers who can sit with your loved one, but you must request this service. If you can afford it, there may be times that you utilize paid home health aides to care for your loved one. It helps to stay fairly close to home when your loved one seems particularly frail, but there are still activities you can engage in to relieve the stress of hospice care. Go to the local gym, take a long walk in a local park, meet a friend for coffee and conversation -- just leave a phone number where you can be reached in an emergency. You'll feel better knowing that you can be there quickly if there's a problem.

Caregiver Tip – You Need to Make It Work for You And You Alone

This is your support team. It's just for you. Pick the people you think are most likely to help. Recognize what each person can do for you. During hospice care, more than at any other time, you need to have people to share your emotions with, so supportive emails, cards, letters, and calls are important tools that can help you feel connected to life as you watch your loved one moving towards death. You may not be able to leave the home whenever you want, so beef up your connections to the outside world in virtual ways. Help yourself not to feel so alone.

SECTION SEVEN -- ORGANIZE THE MEDICAL CARE IN HOME HOSPICE

The first thing any caregiver benefits from is to review the loved one's health situation. Assess the needs of your loved one, so that you can begin to develop strategies to help your loved one get the best medical care available. In home hospice, the hospice team will come to the home, usually on an as-needed basis. The hospice team will rely on you to provide accurate observations and information on your loved one's condition.

1. Medications – You are the official pharmacy assistant.

In hospice, the hospice team will provide the medications you will need to keep your loved one as comfortable as possible. Many of these drugs are very powerful – some are controlled substances, such as morphine. Medication management is important in hospice caregiving. You need to understand the drugs you are providing, the dosages, and the times to give the medications. Some medicines are time-release or slow-acting. Some are quick-release and short-acting. Sitting down with your hospice team and going over each medication and how it works can help you avoid making critical mistakes.

2. Medical History – You are the official medical coordinator.

Generally speaking, by the time your loved one needs hospice care, there is significant reason to believe that cure is no longer an option. The hospice team may ask you for information on your loved one's medical history during the initial visit. If you have records, you can share these. But once your loved one begins hospice care, his or her medical history may not play a role in hospice care, unless it creates a complication. You will be expected to update the hospice team on any issues or physical conditions as they occur, in order to address them in the most effective manner possible, to insure your loved one's comfort.

3. Issues and Complications – You are the official chief information officer.

By the time your loved one needs hospice care, he or she also usually needs a full-time caregiver. Generally speaking, your loved one will be treated only for complications that cause discomfort or distress. Some hospice patients occasionally need emergency hospital care or, when things are too precarious, a transfer to a medical hospice. Check with your hospice team before you call 911. This is especially important if your loved one has a Do Not Resuscitate order. Remember, you're not trying to cure your loved one's illness any more. But occasionally, things happen and your loved one needs medical attention. For example, if there is an infection, your loved one may be treated with antibiotics. This doesn't change the fact that your loved one is still moving towards death, nor will it prevent the natural course of death from occurring, but it may make your loved one feel more comfortable. In some cases, lab tests may be ordered. Some tests require your loved one to prepare ahead of time. Many medical laboratories have technicians that will come to the house to test your loved one. Be sure you understand all instructions, including any regarding fasting, taking required dyes, and medications. If you have questions, always call the laboratory or physician's office to double-check.

4. Nutrition and Diet – You are the official

nutrition coordinator.

If you are a long-time family caregiver, you will see some very big changes when your loved one enters a hospice program. His or her appetite is likely to change significantly. Discuss this with the hospice team, so that you understand these changes. Make a list of all nutritional information that is important for your loved one. What kinds of foods will be palatable to your loved one? When should you worry that your loved one is not eating? Some medications must be taken with food and if your loved one is not eating, it can create serious problems. Your hospice team will tell you what to do in these circumstances.

Food can be an issue that creates power struggles between patient and caregiver if it's not properly addressed. Some hospice caregivers insist that a loved one eat, no matter what. Your job is to meet the *real* needs of your loved one. Dying patients lose their appetites because their bodies are breaking down as they move towards death. Their bodies can no longer process food successfully. Always seek nutritional advice from medical professionals, dietitians, and nutritionists on how best to help your loved one. If you find yourself upset by your loved one's refusal to eat, talk to your hospice team. You need support and education to handle the stress that can result from the realization that your loved one is no longer interested in eating because he or she is dying.

Caregiver Tip – Comfort and Compassion Help Your Loved One Find Peace at the End of Life

Home hospice care is often very stressful, because things can constantly change. Your loved one may have good days and bad days. Don't neglect the emotional and mental aspects of home hospice care. Ask yourself what's more important at that moment in time -- to take care of that load of laundry or to emotionally connect with your loved one. Why not sit down with a cup of coffee or tea and relax for a few minutes with your loved one? When you really need to take care of physical responsibilities, you may ask a family member to sit with your loved one. Hospice care is comfort care and just having someone there can sometimes be reassuring to your loved one.

SECTION EIGHT -- DURING END-OF-LIFE CARE (HOSPICE)

What you can expect:

-- You are likely to provide and/or coordinate around-the-clock caregiving

-- The hospice team comes to the home to provide medical treatment and to instruct you in care

-- You, as the family caregiver, work with the hospice team

-- This is a very emotional time for family and friends

-- Directed comfort care and pain management can ease suffering for your loved one

-- There are often rapid physical changes, and medical treatment is likely to change with each

-- Rest is important for your loved one and you may see a significant increase in sleeping

Common Tasks in End-of-Life Care:

-- You are the hospice coordinator, working under the direction of the hospice team

-- Your goal is provide your loved one with the best comfort care possible

-- Medication and nutrition management for the dying patient are critical

-- You are likely to provide physical assistance for most or all activities

-- You can help loved one finish unfinished business

-- You are likely to keep family and friends directly informed of loved one's condition, or work with a family member to do so

Common Issues in End-of-Life Care:

-- Many families experience depression, anger, sadness during hospice care

-- Your loved one may feel frustration with or

denial of impending death

-- He or she may have fears of how death will come and what will happen to the family afterwards

-- The family may feel uncertainty and dread as your loved one's health begins to spiral downward

-- Your loved one may have extreme fatigue due to the physicality of death

-- Physical pain, discomfort and muscle atrophy may result from the body's deterioration

-- In preparing for death, your love one may physically and socially withdraw

Caregiver Goals in End-of-Life Care:

-- Provide physical, mental, and emotional comfort

-- Coordinate with the hospice team and family

-- Take respite time, especially because you need to accept the reality of hospice care

-- Accept that the death of your loved one is not a failure of your care

When the End Comes....

-- Gather your family and friends together

-- Understand that your emotions will be strong

-- Reach out to each other and share your grief and your memories

-- Honor your loved one

PART TWO: THE HEART AND SOUL OF HOSPICE

SECTION NINE -- HOSPICE IS END-OF-LIFE CAREGIVING

Frustrated Fran takes her father home from the hospital after the physician suggests it is time for him to enter a hospice program. She decides to get a second and then a third opinion, because she is sure there is a cure out there for his damaged heart. While she is running around, looking for new treatments, her father spends his last days trying to please his daughter, instead of finishing up his final "to do" list and saying his goodbyes.

Forlorn Felicia takes her father home from the hospital after the physician suggests it is time for him to enter a hospice program. She spends some time reading up on the concept of hospice, so she understands how to help her father. They spend many afternoons going through his personal papers, writing letters to old friends, planning his funeral and obituary, and playing cards. Forlorn Felicia invites family to visit, so they can spend time with him before he dies. Sometimes they just sit together, watching TV, while her father dozes in his chair.

Frustrated Fran refuses to accept the fact that her father is now struggling with daily living. She ignores the reality that his breathing is labored, he's lost a considerable amount of weight, and he has trouble walking more than just a couple feet. When she looks at him, she doesn't see that this once-strapping man is now shrunken, his muscles wasting away. Fran wants what she wants, for her father to live forever, and she's not willing to force herself out of denial in order to provide her father with the comfort he needs in his last days.

Forlorn Felicia, on the other hand, may be sad at the prospect of saying goodbye to her father, but at the same time, she's trying to pull things together and give her father what he really needs, a peaceful death. It's not that she has given up and raised the white flag of surrender, tossing her father to the wolves. It's that she's seen the physical changes he's experienced and she realizes there's no real chance he can continue living in his broken down body.

Home hospice is an important time for families. It's a chance to make the most of the opportunities to finish unfinished business, to say the final goodbye to someone you love. The more you know and understand about home hospice care, the better the care you will provide. Once you accept that you cannot make your loved one better, you can focus on making him or her feel better. Comfort is the key to success in home hospice care.

Not all hospice patients have the same experience. Some continue to live a mostly normal life, right up to the end. Some have a hard struggle because of the nature of their complicated health challenges. And the rest seem to fall somewhere in between, often having good days up until the last week or two. As caregivers, we don't always know what's going to happen until it happens.

Good hospice care is flexible, adapting your efforts to meet the rapidly changing needs of your loved one. What works for one person won't work for another. We don't all share the same "Bucket list".

Many hospice patients have limited activities outside the home. But many hospice patients still enjoy sitting outside on a nice afternoon when it's feasible or even going for a ride. I remember a visit to a hospice by the sea. I was very impressed by the fact that so many dying patients had the chance to be wheeled outside on a summer's day. They were able to listen to the waves roll in and hear the gulls call to one another. Listen to your loved one and do what you can to accommodate his or her wishes.

One of the biggest responsibilities for hospice caregivers is medication management. It's important to keep track of what is taken and when it is taken. You can also do this the old-fashioned way, using a paper notebook, recording the time and dosage of the medication, or with an app. When you're stressed (a common occurrence for hospice caregivers), it's easy to forget to dispense this pill or that capsule. By recording the medications and the time you dispense them, you guarantee that errors are minimized. You can also note new or recurring symptoms that you observe. Share this information with the hospice team, in order to better meet your loved one's needs. Sometimes there are better alternatives to the prescribed medications.

If your loved one is physically uncomfortable or experiencing pain, panic, or anxiety, work with the hospice team to resolve the problem. No hospice patient should be in agony. Palliative care physicians understand how to medicate people who are experiencing specific types of discomfort. Your loved one deserves to have symptoms properly managed.

There may also be some issues that will surface after your loved one's death. Having a record of what happened during hospice may be helpful. It's also a way to remember what your loved one experienced while in hospice.

Caregiver tip – start (or restart) yourself off on the right foot

Some family caregivers can find the challenges of home hospice care to be nearly impossible, especially if there aren't a lot of family members, friends, or neighbors available to help, or if the physical demands of caregiving are more than they can provide. It's important to be creative in finding the kinds of resources that can help you get through it. Talk to your family, friends, and the hospice team to find reasonable solutions.

PART THREE: HEADING TOWARD DEATH

SECTION TEN -- THE DYING PROCESS CHANGES EVERYTHING

Sad Sammy wants to make his Uncle Danny as comfortable as possible while he's in hospice. He changes Uncle Danny's double bed for a motorized hospital bed, kicks Scruffy the Cat out, and puts a "do not disturb" sign on his uncle's bedroom door. Everyone is instructed to tiptoe and whisper, so as to not bother Uncle Danny. The only trouble is Uncle Danny's not quite ready to die yet. Boy, it's going to be a long two months....

Sorrowful Sid wants to make his Uncle Mort as comfortable as possible while he's in hospice. He sits down with his uncle to discuss what the dying man wants done. They decide to keep Uncle Mort's double bed as long as possible -- it's the one he shared with Aunt Junie for so long. Uncle Mort wants Screech the Cat to come and go as he pleases. He also wants to know what will happen to his pet after his death. Sorrowful Sid promises to take care of the old flea bag. He also puts an arm chair in Uncle Mort's room, so family and friends can keep him company while he rests.

Sad Sammy and Sorrowful Sid both want what's best for their uncles, but Sid doesn't presume to know what his uncle is going through. He's willing to have a dialogue. For someone like Uncle Mort, there's great comfort in remaining with the familiar and comforting memories of home. Keeping that bed he shared with his late wife as long as possible is important to him, just like making plans for Screech is. Many pet owners have real concerns about what happens to their loyal companions after they die. If you're not an animal person, you might think it's no big deal. Talk to folks who do animal rescue -- they can tell you how many beloved pets are given up for adoption because no arrangements were made. Even if he can't take the cat, Sid knows he's responsible for making sure Screech has a good home.

Both Uncle Danny and Uncle Mort have concerns as their lives draw to a close. They also have limited time and energy. That's why it's so critical to focus on what our loved ones want to do with the time they have left.

If you are new to the hospice situation, it's important for you to understand how the caregiver structure is evolving. In order to enter a hospice program, patients normally have to fit the specific criteria. That means there are physical signs that the body has begun to break down and there is little likelihood this damage can be reversed. A well-meaning caregiver might to try to "fix" the patient, by seeking a cure, but it's often a waste of time. This can result in the patient frittering away those valuable remaining weeks and months undergoing painful procedures and enduring discomfort from useless treatments. Studies have shown that patients in hospice programs often live longer and better than those who continue to actively pursue a cure.

Every human being needs to feel that life is worth living right up to that last breath. With a supportive family that's willing to take on the physical challenges, our loved ones can find peace. How do we make that happen? We do it by recognizing those who are dying often have unmet needs and unfulfilled dreams.

For example, Pop might want to take everyone to Disney World, but we know he just doesn't have the strength to make the journey. If we think about why he wants that dream, we can begin to understand what's behind the desire -- a chance to bring the family together for some special memories. Once the family understands what Pop's hoping to achieve with an impractical trip to Disney World, they can give him what he really needs -- the family getting together for some fun. Pop's caregiver might arrange for family members to regularly visit him. Why not turn the house into a mini-version of Disney World? Maybe everyone gets a pair of mouse ears to wear. Maybe the grandkids get dressed up as Disney characters and have their photos taken with Pop. The family might arrange for a virtual trip to Disneyland, thanks to videos, games, and even travel shows, gathering together to play and have fun together. After all, that's really what Pop wants, isn't it? He wants to hear the grandkids giggle and see his kids laughing. Most of all, he wants to share it with his wife one last time.

Patients who have accepted the terminal nature of their disease are often willing to discuss the situation with their families. Sometimes, however, when there are still unresolved issues, they are not. It's not the responsibility of any caregiver to inform a loved one that death is imminently hovering on the horizon; nor is it a caregiver's responsibility to tell a loved one to let go, or that it's time to die. Imagine how you would feel being shoved out the Door of Life by a pushy relative.

Instead, you can focus on getting to the heart of what matters most to your loved one. "How can I help you? What would you like me to do for you?" Comfort, compassion, and good listening skills are the best tools for home hospice caregivers. The whole concept of a peaceful death is about helping a loved one to feel free to let go of the mortal coil when it's time. Sometimes the biggest problem our loved ones have is that their unspoken regrets hold them back, weighing heavily on their minds because they carry a sense of guilt that they somehow failed us by not being cured. When caregivers keep the lines of communication open, our loved ones often reach out to us to share those thoughts that trouble them, in the hopes we will help them find the comfort they seek.

Your role shifts from being proactive and focused on cure to helping your loved one get ready for that final journey. Make a list of the things your loved one wants and needs to do to prepare for death. If there is an interest in sharing final wishes, thoughts, and directives, record them -- on paper, as an audio file, or on video; if your loved one has the stamina, you might even get creative and put it into book form, as a lasting legacy to the family. Discuss activities your loved one wants to undertake. Does he want to plan his own funeral? Does she want to record some favorite stories for her children or grandchildren to remember her by? Does he want to write letters to people he loves, to share his final thoughts on how much they mean to him? Does she want to throw out personal papers or keep them, assigning a specific family member to receive them? Finishing the final "to do" list can be tiring. Take the time to observe your loved one as you work together. When it becomes emotionally overwhelming, take a step back. Let your loved one decide what gets done. You're there to help.

Your presence can be comforting to your loved one, even if you just sit quietly and work on a puzzle or read a book in the same room. Remind yourself of this when you feel like all you do is run around. Give yourself permission to stop and take a breather. People who are dying can feel lonely when their caregivers are so busy that they can't take a break for a cup of tea or to just relax. Don't spend all your time "doing" for your loved one. Don't rush off to "get back to work". Make time to be a companion.

Now, more than ever, you are the official skills optimizer. Make a list of the things your loved one can do by himself or herself at this moment in time. These can be used to maintain a sense of self-worth in your loved one, even during hospice. Find ways to enable him or her to continue achieving. Let your loved one's voice be heard, whether it's to impart wisdom to the family or share stories of days gone by. Ask if you can record the conversations, either with audio or video, or write them down.

You are still the official social coordinator, but now you will have to be cognizant of your loved one's growing limitations and fading energy. Many hospice patients can still participate in activities, so consider what is possible for your loved one. You may still get together for family gatherings, but keep it simple. Friends and neighbors may still come by, but only if your loved one agrees it's a positive experience.

Don't be surprised when you and other family members have a hard time coping with your emotions. Being so close to a dying person often triggers reactions. We see a person we love lying in a bed, and as death comes closer, he or she begins to leave us. Little by little, the person we knew disappears. That is often heartbreaking. You all need to process your feelings and find strength in your support for each other. Call the social worker or chaplain if you or a family member is struggling to cope.

One of the biggest adjustments in hospice for a caregiver comes at mealtime. You're not likely to sit down with your loved one to eat anymore. You may be tempted to skip meals or to wolf down sweets. Be aware that you need to maintain a nutritious diet to continue caring for your loved one.

Make sure you have access to healthy foods and snacks. You need to be alert, especially in the later stages of hospice. If your appetite is affected (it happens to the best of us), focus on foods that are quick and easy to get down -- soup, scrambled eggs, peanut butter-and-jelly sandwiches, yogurt, even nutritional shakes and hot cocoa.

One can be a very lonely number when you're on your own for dinner. Don't be afraid to reach out to others and ask them to keep you company. Your supporters are more than willing to bring a meal and share it with you, so invite them in.

Pop quiz: Your loved one is sleeping in the recliner while you watch TV. What's the best choice of program?

A. "Texas Chainsaw Massacre" -- your loved one won't mind if you watch it because he's sleeping anyway

B. "The Godfather" -- the musical score is lovely and it's all about family

C. Anything you want, as long as you use ear buds

Imagine trying to sleep while terrified screams fill the air. What could be worse than that? Try the whirring of power saws to accompany the "No! Please don't kill me!" pleas of the victims. The theme from "The Godfather" is instantly recognizable; so is the dialogue when Marlon Brando does that cotton-in-the-mouth speech. Does your loved one really need to think about a horse head left in bed or who's going to get whacked next? With ear buds on, you're the only one who can hear the hum of the power saw or the rat-a-tat-tat of the machine gun, so you're free to pick the scariest movie you can find, (although I don't recommend it before you go to bed.)

As a caregiver, you have some measure of control over the noises your loved one is subjected to during hospice. If you've ever spent time with a hospitalized patient, you probably know that it can be irritating for someone trying to sleep to be subjected to endless conversations, constant banging and beeping, and especially the unexpected slamming of a door. Try to err on the side of quiet if your loved one isn't participating in the activity. The goal here is to protect your loved one from noise that can trigger unpleasant nightmares or disrupt sleep.

PART FOUR: THE TOLL OF HOSPICE CAREGIVING

SECTION ELEVEN -- HOSPICE CAREGIVING CAN AFFECT YOU

Stress, depression, and physical neglect can have a negative impact on you, especially if you are working around the clock. You need to be able to focus, to manage crises that arise, and to meet the constantly changing demands of caregiving. That requires you to take good care of yourself, so you will be able to be there for your loved one. Unless you're stranded on a desert island with your loved one, you should never do hospice caregiving all by yourself. It's too much for any human being to take on. You need to know who you can call on for those times you need help. A good caregiver support team will help you avoid some of the biggest pitfalls of taking care of a loved one at the end of life.

Some caregivers get creative with their lists. For

example, there's no reason why you can't ask your neighbor, Kathy, if she can pick up a gallon of milk, a dozen eggs, a loaf of bread, and some gelato from the store. You know she's said several times she'd like to help you. And if your brother, Dean, isn't exactly handy around the house or good at changing bed sheets, don't count him out. Ask him to spend an hour visiting with your father while you get some household chores done. Need some fresh air? Ask your father's buddy, Ronnie, to spend some time sitting with him while you get outside and take a long walk.

Feel too guilty to ask folks for help? Would you feel better if it actually was a positive thing for your loved one? Consider this, when Kathy gets you those groceries, you won't waste time fretting about how you can be in two places at once. That means you'll be calmer around your loved one, and he won't have to deal with your anxiety. Dean and your father benefit from having a chance to strengthen their bond; it's a chance for Dean to be compassionate and a time for your dad to share important thoughts, should he desire. They might just take a trip down Memory Lane and talk about favorite experiences, like the ball games they went to at Yankee Stadium. And as for Ronnie and your dad, well...what buddy would mind keeping company with a true and loyal friend? Even if

Ronnie just sits there, saying nothing, that camaraderie counts. See, caregiver? It's not selfish on your part to call in the troops. It's a win-win-win.

Your loved one shouldn't be left alone at home while in hospice care, especially when he or she can no longer stand without assistance. That's because the risk of falling is very high. The last thing your loved one needs is broken bones or a traumatic brain injury. It's important that everyone who shares the care for your loved one understands this.

It's inevitable that you will shed tears during hospice and find yourself grappling with your emotions as you begin to see signs that death is coming. You need a shoulder or two to cry on, but not just any shoulder. The harder the challenges you face, the greater the need for quality support. You will benefit from having good people who can listen to you vent when frustrations and sadness get the better of you, and offer you wise counsel on everything from family conflicts to medical mess-ups to ordinary mole hills that might become mountains if you don't knock them down to size.

Being a hospice caregiver can be a lonely role, especially in the wee, small hours of the night. The fear, the sheer terror of being with a dying person can take its toll. It's important to know that you can connect with other people who can ease that pain you bear. I've found that having the chance to text, both as a caregiver and as a caregiver supporter, can offer real-time support for those tenuous times. When someone is in need of a kind word or encouragement to get through the crisis, whether it's physical, emotional, or even spiritual, it matters. Camaraderie is important for hospice caregivers because you're often isolated from the rest of the world as your loved one is dying.

If you have good friends or compassionate relatives who live far away, don't leave them out of your hospice circle. People who live in a different time zone are often the people who are available when you're feeling blue or desperate. These are often the people who will keep you going with their virtual companionship. It's nice to know people are there for you, ready to hear you out.

And believe it or not, you might be amazed by how good it is, when you've got a plateful of grief on your table, to listen to someone you know describe normal, everyday problems going on at the other end of the conversation. Suddenly, you're not a hospice caregiver stuck at home. You're back to being a person in the "real" world, where ordinary things happen to ordinary people. It's a reminder to you that someday you will be back in that same position, fielding life's tiny annoyances, rather than carrying this heavy burden you bear as you care for your dying loved one.

Pop quiz: If you do everything right during hospice, what's likely to happen?

A. It will be sunshine, lollipops, and rainbows all the way

B. Your loved one will get better

C. You will have ups and downs, laughter and tears, and you'll learn things about your loved one that you never knew

If you're hoping there will be sunshine, lollipops, and rainbows in hospice, you're certainly an optimist. Did you forget the part about the rain? While there is the occasional situation in which a person improves enough to move out of hospice for a while, before health declines again, it's very rare. And yet, despite the challenges, hospice can be a positive experience, especially when you know you've done right by your loved one.

There's not a caregiver alive who hasn't dreaded the end of a loved one's life, so you might think there's nothing wonderful about hospice. But in reality, those little moments of clarity and understanding that grow out of the still-evolving relationship between loved ones and caregivers make it all worthwhile somehow.

PART FIVE: AS THE END NEARS

SECTION TWELVE -- DON'T BE ALONE WHEN YOUR LOVED ONE DIES

The average caregiver has little or no experience with dead bodies, so it's hard to imagine what it will happen when your loved one passes away. Depending on the hospice program you use, you may have a paid or volunteer assistant to help you with some of the physical tasks involved in the hours just before death. If your loved one has pain or needs to be turned for comfort purposes, it helps to have someone there to share the task. My own experience has taught me that it's good not to be alone. It helps to talk to another human being, to feel connected to other people. Very often, towards the end of life, family members and supportive friends hold a vigil. We sit and talk. We might play favorite music to comfort us. We might look out for each other. Often the most important thing we can do is be there at our loved one's side, for that last touch, that final farewell. But when death finally comes, what happens next?

People react in their own ways at the end of hospice. They may be sad, angry, stunned, stoic, or even relieved that a loved one's suffering has now ended. What comes next?

In most cases, the caregiver calls the hospice team to announce that death has occurred. A nurse usually comes to the house to fill out the death certificate and to help organize the removal of the body. Will there be a funeral? This is something that is often arranged while the loved one is in the final days of life. Some families, especially when a loved one has been ill for a while, or if the care has been particularly difficult, will opt to skip the funeral and hold a memorial service at a later date. Other families need that support in the days following death and have a full funeral. It helps to give this some thought ahead of time. If your loved one has expressed a particular desire, do what you can to honor that request.

As terrible as it might seem, the more you can plan ahead and make arrangements, the better. Will there be an open casket? Will your loved one be cremated? Will you invite people back to the house for a gathering or opt for a light meal at a restaurant or banquet facility? Who will officiate at the service? Who will speak? Most important of all, what is the budget for the final farewell? Believe it or not, taking these steps helps you to adjust to the reality that your loved one really is about to die.

But when death comes, what is it like? And what is it like to be with a dead body? Some people want nothing to do with the dead body. Some people are reluctant to let the funeral home workers remove it. Much of your reaction to death is tied in with your religious and spiritual beliefs, your views on illness, your ability to cope with the stress of both hospice caregiving and the loss of your loved one, and also your level of exhaustion at that moment in time. There is no one right answer. People need to do what they have to do in their own way and in their own time. I've known people who, in the last hours of life, had to excuse themselves from the hospice setting because they couldn't handle it. I've also known people who needed to be able to sit for a few hours with their deceased loved ones. It's a way of reassuring yourself your loved one is actually gone. As the skin cools and the color changes, your mind begins to absorb the fact that it's really finally over. You come to grips with the fact that your loved one really has departed. Your brain and your heart are trying to reconcile the new reality. Your mind has to wrap around the fact that death is permanent. Your heart has to find a way to cope with all the pain it feels.

Caregiver tip: Be Careful about Announcing Your Loved One's Death Publicly

We had a very unfortunate experience after a loved one's death. While relatives were still in the process of contacting family members with the news, it was posted on social media and the news quickly was circulated. Imagine having a close relative learn of a loved one's passing this way. It was devastating. The person who made the public announcement had good intentions. It was supposed to be a kind gesture. But there was no way for him to know what the family was doing. Thus, have a plan for who to contact and make sure that those people who need to be informed personally have that news before it goes public.

PART SIX: AFTER THE CAREGIVING

SECTION THIRTEEN -- GRIEF AND GRIEVING

In this updated edition of my hospice guide, I decided to offer some suggestions for those who are grieving. It came as the result of a friend reaching out to me for help in comforting an exhausted caregiver who had some post traumatic stress after a grueling experience providing hospice care. I knew exactly why it was important. It's hard to turn off our caregiver mindset after we've been at it all day and all night. We throw ourselves into our caregiving because we know how critical it is to get it right. There is no do-over for death.

I've found again and again that when a loved one is finally gone, coping with all the raw emotions can seem overwhelming. If you've been providing intensive care around the clock, the first few days, weeks, and even months after loss can be extremely lonely. Your purpose for being a caregiver is gone. How do you fill all those hours?

My secret is this. Know what makes you feel connected, not only to life, but also to your loved one. It's okay to cry when you remember. It helps to talk to other people who also loved him or her. But above all, find a healthy physical release.

When my mom died, I hiked miles and miles through the woods. I needed to be surrounded by nature. It was something I had done on my respite time as a caregiver. I would often take photographs to show her of my adventures.

When my brother died, I worked in his garden. I raked leaves, pruned tree branches, and rebuild parts of his beloved stone walls. It helped me to get used to the idea that he wasn't coming back to the place he loved so much. With every swipe of the rake, I thought of him. With every snip of the pruning shears, I thought of him. With every boulder I moved, I thought of him.

But it had another positive effect. It gave me a chance to connect with my sister-in-law. It gave us both a healthy outlet for all the tears, the sorrow.

Sorrow is an unavoidable part of the grieving process. It will hit you when you least expect it. For me, driving by the trails my brother and I both loved made me sad. Looking out at the lake he loved made me sad. It's like the words of that old Sammy Fain and Irving Kahal song:

I'll be seeing you in all the old familiar places

That this heart of mine embraces all day through

In that small cafe, the park across the way

The children's carousel, the chestnut tree, the wishing well....

You will remember the sights and sounds of your loved one. It's the ordinary, everyday memories that seem to follow us everywhere we go after death. Those normal activities we shared when our loved ones were still able seem harder to embrace when we're alone.

And yet, you will find that sometimes you just have to find comfort in the familiar. I still enjoy going down to the river, where my mom and I used to picnic. After my mom's health declined to the point she was housebound, I sometimes managed to convince her to get in the car and ride with me to the river. She would walk ten steps to the picnic table and collapse, her oxygen tank at her side, for a picnic lunch. For that short hour, she could forget her pain and enjoy being outdoors again. It was her way of feeling free, even as her health deteriorated. It was a place she enjoyed being, and so when I am there, I can remember happier times.

As sad as it is to know that a loved one has passed, it helps to remember the joy we shared. In the first year, grief will seem to catch you at the heels and yank you to the ground, despite your best efforts to remain standing. What can you do to keep yourself going? Know what you can handle and what you can't. Be honest with yourself, because that will help you take positive steps during your bereavement.

PART SEVEN: THE EMPTY CHAIR

SECTION FOURTEEN -- COPING WITH THE LOSS

It helps to adjust your expectations for family celebrations after a loved one dies. When you look at that empty chair, all you can think about is what you no longer have. The tendency is to forget what you still have because you're so aware of who's missing.

1. Do "Un-Holidays"

Changing the usual menus, the normal seating arrangements, the time you gather with family, or any other detail that will help you get through the celebration. Make it deliberately different, to let yourself adjust.

2. Serve comfort food

The thought of preparing meals after the loss of a loved one was particularly challenging for me. It seemed to force us back into the past in a way that only made us overly aware that our loved one wasn't with us. But comfort food is comfort food. It goes down easy. It is simple and plain. It is family friendly. For several holidays, I made a big side dish of macaroni and cheese. It was normally the first thing to go. I stopped worrying about doing things "the traditional way". I tossed out the rules and focused on helping family members reconnect.

3. Respect the fact that everyone has a different comfort level and different ways of coming to terms with death

You may find other people expect you to "get over it" within a set period of time. But grief comes in stages, and we don't all go through each stage the same way. Listen to your heart and your head. Know that you have to be able to function in the here-and-now and in the future. You can't stay locked in your past with your loved one. You need to find a way to integrate your past with your loved one with your new life.

4. Good grieving takes time

Forcing yourself to move forward before you have adjusted to the loss of your loved one can have negative consequences for you and the people around you. If you rush through the process, you may miss important healing steps.

5. You will have good days and bad days

It's a given that you will have times that are emotionally challenging and charged, but as the days and weeks pass, there is likely to be an ebb and flow of sorrow. The trick is to get through the low points, so that you can be there for the better moments. You do that by moving forward with baby steps. Do what feels right to you.

6. Beware of becoming stuck on what went wrong

Often those who need hospice have been dealing with serious health challenges over a long period of time, whether it's cancer, COPD, heart disease, or any of a number of diseases and illnesses. For many caregivers, it's easy to get stuck in what could have been or what should have been, in the face of what was. It hurts to think about how life might have been changed by a diagnosis found sooner, a medical treatment not taken, or a different action you might have tried. Life is not a do-over. All we can do as caregivers is to do the best we can in every moment we provide care. And once that care ends, we need to recognize that we are human. We may not have been perfect in every act, but we gave it our best. That's all anyone can expect of us.

7. Our loved ones know we wanted what was best for them

In those moments when you have frustrations or doubts about what happened to your loved one as hospice became necessary, it helps to remind yourself that you really did have their best interests in mind.

8. Our loved ones want us to have what is best for us

Relationships that are built on love and trust forge important bonds. When you feel overwhelmed, ask yourself what your loved one would want for you. Would he or she want you to be miserable, or would he or she want you to have a good life? When you pose this question to yourself, give it some serious thought. Really try to see what your loved one's perspective would be. Just as you wanted your loved one to have a full, happy life, that's what he or she would want for you now.

9. Be patient with yourself

Don't beat yourself up when you stumble or fall. Pick yourself up and slow down to a pace you can maintain. Grief is like a marathon. There will be peaks and valleys. Reserve some energy for those challenging hills and coast when you've got the chance. Steady really does get you to where you need to be.

Finally, don't be afraid to get help if you need it. Reach out to friends and family. Join a bereavement group and talk to others who have similar experiences. Do things that help to reduce your loneliness. You are now an experienced caregiver; you did a good job caring for your loved one. Now it's time to turn those skills to your need for care. Be a good caregiver for yourself. That is what your loved one would want for you, and by taking good care of yourself, you complete the final task of any good hospice caregiver. You point yourself in the right direction. You carry the love with you as you begin the next chapter of your life. Make it count. That's how you honor your loved one.

ABOUT THE AUTHOR

Sara M. Barton, who trained as an educator, interacted with hospitalized children during her first teaching practicum in the pediatric department of a large city hospital, gaining insight into the value of play therapy and socialization during medical treatment. With minors in art and psychology, she later worked with adult patients in a psychiatric admissions hospital and disturbed adolescents in residential care. These experiences were invaluable when caring for her mother over more than a decade. She created the Practical Caregiver Guides website and Practical Caregiver blogs to help family caregivers:

Practical Caregiver Guides Website for Family Caregivers:

https://practicalcaregiverguides.org

Sara M. Barton is the author of several fast-paced cozy mysteries featuring lively characters: *The Scarlet Wilson Mysteries, The Off the Books Mysteries, The International Killer Chefs Competition Mysteries* (The first book in the new series is entitled *Frosted!*)

She has also written hybrid "cozy thriller" series, offering likeable characters and wild twists: *The*

Gabby Grimm Fairy Tale Mysteries, The Cornwall & Company Mysteries

She also has written dark and dangerous spy thrillers based on historical events dating back to the Cold War. Some of these touch on now-unclassified government-funded research programs examining the feasibility of psychic abilities: *The Project Stargazer Thrillers, The Arden Woods Thrillers*

Sara Barton Mysteries:

https://smbarton.com

www.ingramcontent.com/pod-product-compliance
Lightning Source LLC
Chambersburg PA
CBHW061157180526
45170CB00002B/844